WHERE ARE MEN?

AN OUTCRY OF GENDER- BASED VIOLENCE AGAINST WOMEN AND CHILDREN IN SOUTH AFRICA

MICHAEL MOKOBANE

First Edition 2024

Published by Michael Mokobane

Introduction

Gender-based violence (GBV) against women and children in South Africa is more than a pressing issue; it is a crisis that affects the very core of our communities. Despite the strides we have made in laws and awareness, the reality is stark: the levels of violence remain devastatingly high, shattering the lives of countless individuals and families.

This book, "Where Are Men? An Outcry of Gender-Based Violence against Women and Children in South Africa," is not just about exploring the depth of this problem. It's a heartfelt call to action. By diving into the historical, cultural, and societal layers that fuel GBV, it aims to uncover the roots of this enduring crisis and its far-reaching effects. More importantly, it shines a spotlight on the voices of survivors, giving them the space to share their experiences and be heard.

The book also highlights the crucial role men must play in addressing this issue. Men are not just bystanders; they are key to both perpetuating and dismantling the cycle of violence. It's essential for men to recognize their part in this fight and actively contribute to building a safer, fairer society.

"Where Are Men?" encourages readers to reflect deeply on their own attitudes and behaviours. It challenges them to confront and change harmful norms and to join the broader movement against GBV. The path to a violence-free society is long and demanding, but every effort counts. This book is a step towards that vision, a plea for change, and a call for justice.

Contents

CHAPTER 1: INTRODUCTION TO GENDER-BASED VIOLENCE IN SOUTH AFRICA

The Scope of the Crisis

Gender-based violence (GBV) in South Africa is a deeply troubling issue that cuts across all sections of society but hits women and children the hardest. Even with laws in place and growing public awareness, the reality remains grim. The statistics are stark: one in five women in South Africa faces physical violence from a partner, and the country is among the highest in the world for rates of rape. In 2019 alone, over 42,000 cases of rape were reported, though this number probably falls short of the actual figures due to underreporting and the stigma surrounding these crimes.

The heart-breaking murder of Uyinene Mrwetyana, a University of Cape Town student, in 2019 brought the issue into the spotlight. Her tragic death led to a wave of protests and a renewed demand for action, highlighting the severe and often deadly impact of GBV. These high-profile cases remind us of the urgent need to confront this crisis head-on and to provide meaningful support for those affected.

Historical Context

The ongoing issue of gender-based violence (GBV) in South Africa is deeply rooted in the country's historical, cultural, and social landscape. The legacy of apartheid, with its systemic violence and profound inequality, has fostered an environment where violence is sadly normalized. During apartheid, violence was a pervasive method used to enforce racial segregation and oppression, and its impact continues to shape societal attitudes and behaviours toward violence today.

Cultural norms and gender stereotypes play a significant role in perpetuating GBV. Traditional practices such as lobola (bride price) and ukuthwala (the abduction of young girls for marriage) reinforce outdated and harmful views of women as possessions rather than individuals with rights and autonomy. These practices not only perpetuate male dominance but also create a climate where women may feel compelled to remain silent about abuse, fearing social stigma or retaliation. This cultural backdrop makes it even more challenging for survivors to seek help and escape abusive situations.

Personal Stories

Behind the stark statistics of gender-based violence (GBV) lie deeply personal stories of pain, resilience, and hope. Take Thuli, for instance, a young woman from Soweto whose life has been marked by repeated physical and emotional abuse at the hands of her partner. Despite the severity of the violence she endured, Thuli felt trapped, not only by the abuse but also by economic dependency and societal expectations to keep her family together. It wasn't until she reached out to a local women's shelter that she began to find a way out. With their support and counselling, Thuli started to rebuild her life, finding strength and hope amid the turmoil.

Then there's Zanele, a mother of two from a rural village in the Eastern Cape. For years, she faced relentless abuse from her husband, a situation that also took a heavy toll on her children, who lived in constant fear. Thanks to the intervention of a community-based organization, Zanele found the courage and resources to escape her abusive environment. She and her children were able to find safety and begin the healing process.

These stories are a powerful reminder of the human cost of GBV and underscore the critical need for comprehensive support systems to help survivors rebuild their lives. They highlight the courage and determination of individuals facing unimaginable challenges and the vital role that community support can play in their journey to safety and recovery.

The Need for Urgent Action

The need to tackle gender-based violence (GBV) in South Africa is both urgent and profound. While the country has established important legal protections, such as the Domestic Violence Act and the Sexual Offences Act, the reality is that enforcement often falls short. Law enforcement officers may not always receive adequate training, resources can be scarce, and societal stigma can undermine the effectiveness of these laws. Survivors frequently encounter additional hurdles when seeking help, often facing secondary victimization that can deter them from pursuing justice.

Economic inequality further compounds the problem. Many women find themselves trapped in abusive relationships due to financial dependence on their partners. With limited access to education and job opportunities, escaping such situations becomes even more challenging. Addressing GBV requires a comprehensive approach: strengthening legal protections, improving their enforcement, challenging harmful societal norms, and offering robust support systems for survivors.

Civil society organizations and grassroots movements play an indispensable role in this fight. Groups like POWA (People Opposing Women Abuse), Sonke Gender Justice, and the Rape Crisis Cape Town Trust offer critical services such as counselling, legal aid, and advocacy. Movements like #AmINext and #TotalShutdown have rallied communities, creating powerful platforms for raising awareness and pressuring the government to take more decisive action against GBV.

International support has also been pivotal. Initiatives backed by the United Nations, the European Union, and various non-governmental organizations contribute vital resources and expertise, enhancing local efforts to prevent violence, educate communities, and support survivors. These collaborations help amplify the impact of grassroots work, driving systemic change and offering hope for a future where GBV is no longer a pervasive issue.

Conclusion

Gender-based violence (GBV) in South Africa is both widespread and deeply embedded in our societal fabric. Tackling this crisis calls for a thorough and immediate response. To make progress, we need to grasp the historical backdrop that has shaped this issue, listen to and honour the personal stories of those affected, and recognize the urgent need for action.

Creating a safer and fairer society requires all of us to come together and play our part. Each step, no matter how small, contributes to the broader effort of ending this pervasive violence. The fight against GBV is a shared responsibility, and it's through our collective commitment that we can hope to see real change. Every voice raised, every action taken, and every effort made brings us closer to a world where violence is no longer a daily reality for so many.

CHAPTER 2: UNDERSTANDING THE ROOTSOF GENDER-BASED VIOLENCE

Cultural Factors

Cultural norms and practices have a powerful influence on the perpetuation of gender-based violence (GBV) in South Africa. Traditional beliefs and customs often uphold male dominance and female subordination, creating environments where violence becomes normalized and accepted. Practices like lobola (bride price) and ukuthwala (the abduction of young girls for marriage) are deeply rooted in history and continue to enforce harmful gender norms. For example, lobola can sometimes be seen as a way of asserting ownership over women, undermining their autonomy and reinforcing imbalances in relationships.

In many communities, these cultural and patriarchal values set rigid gender roles, placing women in vulnerable and dependent positions. Such norms can make it difficult for women to speak out against abuse or seek help, as they fear social judgment or exclusion. Meanwhile, traditional views that cast men as protectors and providers, while confining women to submissive roles, can perpetuate cycles of violence. This dynamic discourages men from taking responsibility for their actions and prevents women from asserting their rights, trapping many in a cycle of abuse and silence.

Economic Factors

Economic dependency is a major factor that fuels the prevalence of gender-based violence (GBV) in South Africa. For many women, financial hardship means they are trapped in abusive relationships because they lack the resources to support themselves and their children independently. This dependence on an abuser can make escaping such situations nearly impossible.

The situation is often worsened by limited access to education and job opportunities. Women facing economic struggles are more likely to experience violence because they have fewer options for leaving abusive environments. Additionally, financial instability can increase stress and conflict within households, which can heighten the risk of violence. The lack of economic opportunities creates a vicious cycle where financial dependence keeps women in dangerous situations, making it crucial to address both GBV and economic inequality to create safer environments for all.

Political Factors

Political factors play a significant role in the ongoing prevalence of gender-based violence (GBV) in South Africa. Even though the country has established progressive laws like the Domestic Violence Act and the Sexual Offences Act, the enforcement of these laws can be inconsistent. The effectiveness of these legal protections hinges on strong political will and prioritization of GBV issues, but sometimes political leaders may lack the commitment or resources needed to implement and uphold these measures effectively.

Corruption and inefficiencies within the criminal justice system further complicate the fight against GBV. Survivors often face significant hurdles, such as inadequate support from law enforcement, delays in legal proceedings, and insufficient protection from further harm. These challenges are exacerbated by political instability and shifting priorities, which can divert attention and resources away from sustained efforts to address GBV and support those affected. The result is a system that struggles to provide the necessary protection and justice for survivors, underscoring the need for both political commitment and systemic reform to truly combat GBV.

Psychological Factors

Psychological factors have a profound impact on both the perpetration and experience of gender-based violence (GBV). For those who commit acts of violence, underlying issues such as difficulties with anger management, unresolved childhood trauma, and exposure to violence can significantly influence their behaviour. Many perpetrators have themselves been victims or witnesses of violence, leading them to view abusive behaviour as normal or acceptable.

For survivors, the psychological scars of GBV can be deep and enduring. The trauma from such violence often leads to mental health challenges like depression, anxiety, and post-traumatic stress disorder (PTSD). The stigma surrounding GBV adds another layer of difficulty, causing survivors to feel ashamed and isolated, which can deter them from seeking the help and support they need. The constant fear of retaliation and the emotional strain of living in a state of anxiety only intensify the psychological impact, making the road to recovery even more challenging.

Conclusion

Understanding the roots of gender-based violence (GBV) in South Africa requires looking at a range of factors—cultural, economic, political, and psychological—that contribute to this complex issue. Cultural norms and practices often uphold harmful gender roles and perpetuate violence. For example, traditional beliefs can reinforce male dominance and discourage women from speaking out about abuse. Economic dependency and a lack of resources can trap individuals in abusive situations, making it hard for them to escape.

Political factors also play a crucial role. Inconsistent enforcement of laws and systemic corruption can undermine efforts to combat GBV, leaving survivors without the protection and justice they need. On the psychological front, underlying issues such as trauma and mental health struggles affect both those who commit violence and those who endure it.

To effectively address GBV, we need a comprehensive approach that tackles these root causes. This means challenging harmful cultural norms, improving economic opportunities for women, ensuring laws are enforced consistently, and offering strong support for survivors' mental health. Ending GBV is a challenging journey that requires the combined efforts of individuals, communities, and policymakers. Only by working together can we hope to build a safer, more equitable society.

CHAPTER 3: THE IMPACT ON WOMEN AND CHILDREN

Physical Health Consequences

The physical toll of gender-based violence (GBV) on women and children is both severe and far-reaching. For many survivors, the immediate effects of violence include injuries such as bruises, fractures, and other physical trauma. Beyond these visible injuries, GBV can result in long-term health issues like chronic pain, gastrointestinal problems, and reproductive health complications. Women who face violence are at a higher risk for conditions such as sexually transmitted infections and unwanted pregnancies. Children exposed to violence, either directly or indirectly, may suffer from physical neglect and developmental delays. The physical health consequences of GBV are not only debilitating but also have a profound impact on survivors' overall quality of life.

Mental Health Consequences

The psychological impact of GBV is equally devastating. Survivors often grapple with a range of mental health issues, including depression, anxiety, and post-traumatic stress disorder (PTSD). The trauma experienced can lead to a pervasive sense of fear, helplessness, and worthlessness. For women and children, the effects of such trauma can disrupt their ability to form healthy relationships, maintain employment, and pursue educational opportunities. The stigma associated with GBV can exacerbate these issues, making it difficult for survivors to seek the mental health support they need. The emotional scars left by violence can persist long after the physical wounds have healed, deeply affecting survivors' overall well-being and their ability to lead fulfilling lives.

Economic Impact

The economic ramifications of GBV are significant and far-reaching. Women and children who experience violence often face economic hardships due to the inability to work, loss of income, and increased medical expenses. For many survivors, financial dependency on their abuser can trap them in a cycle of violence, making it challenging to escape. Additionally, the economic impact extends to societal costs, including healthcare expenses, legal fees, and lost productivity. The burden of GBV on the economy is profound, as it undermines the ability of survivors to contribute fully to their communities and to achieve financial independence.

Social Isolation

GBV often leads to profound social isolation for survivors. The fear of stigma and the threat of further violence can push survivors away from their support networks and communities. Women and children facing abuse may withdraw from social interactions, avoid seeking help, and become increasingly isolated. This social withdrawal can further exacerbate feelings of loneliness and helplessness, making it even harder for survivors to find the support they need. Social isolation also limits survivors' access to resources and assistance, making it difficult for them to rebuild their lives and regain their sense of self-worth.

In conclusion, the impact of GBV on women and children extends beyond the immediate effects of violence. It permeates their physical health, mental well-being, economic stability, and social connections. Addressing these impacts requires a holistic approach that not only provides immediate relief but also supports long-term recovery and empowerment. Understanding and acknowledging these consequences is crucial in creating effective strategies to support survivors and prevent future violence.

CHAPTER 4: MEN AS PERPETRATORS

Case Studies

Exploring the role of men as perpetrators of gender-based violence (GBV) requires understanding individual stories and broader patterns. Take, for example, the case of Mark, a middle-aged man from Johannesburg, who was involved in a high-profile domestic violence case. Mark's abusive behaviour stemmed from a combination of unresolved personal issues and a troubling history of witnessing violence in his own childhood. His actions not only devastated his partner but also had a ripple effect on his family and community, highlighting how deeply personal and social factors can intersect in perpetuating violence.

Another case is that of James, a young man from a rural area who was convicted of sexual assault.

James's behaviour was influenced by a lack of education and exposure to harmful gender norms within his community. His case underscores the role that cultural and societal influences play in shaping behaviours and attitudes towards violence. Both Mark and James's stories reveal how personal and societal factors converge to contribute to the prevalence of GBV.

Psychological Profiles

Understanding the psychological profiles of perpetrators can offer insights into the factors driving abusive behaviour. Many men who commit acts of violence have experienced or witnessed violence themselves, leading to a normalization of such behaviour. Issues like unresolved anger, childhood trauma, and poor impulse control can also play significant roles. Perpetrators often have distorted beliefs about power and control, viewing violence as a means to assert dominance or address personal grievances.

Additionally, some perpetrators may struggle with mental health issues that exacerbate their violent behaviour. However, it's crucial to emphasize that while psychological factors can contribute to violence, they do not excuse or justify abusive actions. Recognizing these psychological patterns is essential for developing effective interventions and support systems for both potential perpetrators and survivors.

Societal Influences

Societal influences are pivotal in shaping attitudes and behaviours related to gender-based violence. Cultural norms that perpetuate male dominance and female subordination create environments where violence is often tolerated or even expected. Media portrayals that normalize aggression or depict women as submissive reinforce harmful attitudes and behaviours. Additionally, societal pressures, such as expectations around masculinity, can lead to violence when men feel their masculinity is threatened or undervalued.

Education and community norms also play a significant role. In communities where there is little focus on gender equality and healthy relationships, abusive behaviours are more likely to be perpetuated. Addressing these societal influences involves challenging and changing harmful norms, promoting gender equality, and fostering healthier attitudes towards masculinity and relationships.

Legal Consequences

The legal consequences for men who perpetrate GBV are an important aspect of addressing this issue. While South Africa has robust laws intended to protect survivors and hold perpetrators accountable, the effectiveness of these laws can vary. Inconsistent enforcement, lengthy legal processes, and challenges within the criminal justice system can hinder the pursuit of justice for survivors.

Men who are convicted of GBV face a range of legal repercussions, including imprisonment, fines, and restraining orders. However, the legal process itself can be a significant burden for survivors, who may have to navigate a complex system while dealing with the trauma of violence. Ensuring that legal frameworks are effectively implemented and that perpetrators are held accountable is crucial for both justice and deterrence.

In conclusion, examining men as perpetrators of GBV involves understanding individual cases, psychological profiles, societal influences, and legal consequences. By delving into these aspects, we can gain a deeper understanding of the factors that contribute to violence and work towards more effective prevention and intervention strategies. Addressing these issues requires a multifaceted approach that involves not only legal and psychological support but also societal change and education.

CHAPTER 5: MEN AS VICTIMS

Overlooked Stories

The stories of men who are victims of gender-based violence (GBV) are often overlooked or minimized, overshadowed by more widely discussed issues. Yet, the pain and trauma experienced by these men are real and significant. Take, for instance, the story of David, a young man from Cape Town who endured physical and emotional abuse at the hands of his partner. David's experience was compounded by a lack of understanding and support from those around him, as his suffering was often dismissed or belittled due to prevailing gender norms.

Another poignant story is that of James, an older man who faced severe psychological abuse from a female caregiver. James struggled silently, unable to share his pain due to fear of judgment and a lack of appropriate resources. These stories highlight the silent struggles of male victims, whose experiences often go unnoticed and unaddressed in the broader conversation about GBV.

Societal Stigma

Men who experience GBV often face significant societal stigma, which can prevent them from seeking help and support. Traditional gender norms and expectations can make it difficult for men to admit vulnerability, as there is often a pervasive belief that men should be strong and impervious to abuse. This stigma can lead to feelings of shame, isolation, and confusion, making it challenging for men to come forward and share their experiences.

For instance, the societal expectation that men should be the protectors and not the victims can create a sense of inadequacy and self-blame among male survivors. This stigma not only affects their willingness to seek help but also impacts their mental and emotional well-being, further complicating their path to recovery.

Support Systems

The support systems available for male victims of GBV are often limited and not well publicized. Unlike resources tailored to female survivors, support services for men may not be as accessible or comprehensive. Organizations and helplines specifically catering to male victims are fewer and may lack the visibility needed to reach those in need.

Efforts are being made to address this gap. For example, some organizations are working to create safe spaces for men to share their experiences and seek help without fear of judgment. These support systems can include counselling services, support groups, and educational programs aimed at raising awareness about male victimization and providing appropriate resources.

Path to Healing

Healing from GBV is a complex and individual journey, especially for men who face unique challenges. Acknowledging the trauma, seeking professional help, and finding supportive communities are crucial steps in this process. For men like David and James, finding a therapist who understands the nuances of their experiences and can provide empathetic support is an essential part of healing.

Support groups specifically for male survivors can offer a space to connect with others who have faced similar experiences, providing validation and a sense of solidarity. Additionally, public awareness campaigns can help challenge the stigma surrounding male victimization, encouraging more men to seek help and share their stories.

Ultimately, the path to healing for male victims of GBV involves breaking the silence and stigma, accessing appropriate support, and addressing both the immediate and long-term effects of their experiences. By acknowledging and addressing the needs of male survivors, society can work towards a more inclusive and supportive environment for all victims of violence.

CHAPTER 6: ROLE OF MEDIA IN GENDER-BASED VIOLENCE

Representation in

News

The way gender-based violence (GBV) is represented in the news plays a significant role in shaping public perception and understanding of the issue. Often, news coverage focuses on sensational aspects of violence, highlighting dramatic cases while neglecting the broader, more pervasive nature of GBV. For example, high-profile cases like the murder of a prominent individual might receive extensive media attention, but everyday instances of violence affecting less visible individuals often go unreported.

This focus on sensationalism can contribute to a skewed understanding of GBV, emphasizing extreme cases over systemic issues. Additionally, the portrayal of survivors in the media can sometimes perpetuate harmful stereotypes or portray them as passive victims, rather than active individuals seeking justice and recovery. A more nuanced and empathetic representation in news media is crucial for raising awareness, fostering empathy, and encouraging action to address GBV.

Impact of Social Media

Social media has transformed the landscape of GBV awareness and advocacy. Platforms like X, Facebook, and Instagram have become vital spaces for survivors to share their stories, seek support, and mobilize communities. Hashtags such as #MeToo and #TimesUp have brought global attention to issues of sexual harassment and assault, creating solidarity among survivors and pressuring institutions to take action.

However, social media also has its drawbacks. While it provides a platform for visibility and support, it can also be a space for victim-blaming and harassment. Survivors who speak out may face online abuse or skepticism, which can further traumatize them and discourage others from coming forward. Balancing the positive and negative impacts of social media is essential for creating a supportive environment where survivors feel safe to share their experiences and seek help.

Television and Film

Television and film have a profound influence on cultural perceptions of GBV. These mediums often portray violence in ways that can either perpetuate harmful stereotypes or challenge them. Shows and movies that depict GBV in a realistic and sensitive manner can raise awareness and foster empathy, while those that sensationalize or trivialize violence can reinforce negative attitudes and misconceptions.

For example, a film that explores the complexities of a survivor's experience and their journey towards healing can offer valuable insights and foster understanding. Conversely, a portrayal that glamorizes violence or presents it as a dramatic plot device without addressing its real-life implications can contribute to desensitization and misunderstanding. The media's portrayal of GBV can significantly impact public attitudes and the willingness to address and prevent violence.

Changing the Narrative

Changing the narrative around GBV requires a concerted effort from all sectors of media. It involves moving beyond sensationalism and victim-blaming to present more nuanced and empathetic portrayals of both survivors and perpetrators. Media outlets, filmmakers, and content creators have a responsibility to reflect the realities of GBV accurately and sensitively, promoting a culture of respect and understanding.

Encouraging diverse voices and stories in media representations is key to changing the narrative. Including perspectives from different genders, backgrounds, and experiences can offer a more comprehensive view of GBV and its impact. Media literacy campaigns can also play a role in helping the public critically engage with media portrayals and challenge harmful stereotypes.

In conclusion, the media plays a crucial role in shaping perceptions and conversations about GBV. By improving representation in news, harnessing the power of social media responsibly, and creating thoughtful portrayals in television and film, the media can contribute to a more informed and compassionate society. Changing the narrative around GBV is an ongoing process that requires commitment from media professionals and audiences alike to ensure that stories are told with sensitivity, accuracy, and respect.

CHAPTER 7: LEGAL FRAMEWORKS AND LAW ENFORCEMENT

Existing Laws

South Africa has established several legal frameworks to address gender-based violence (GBV) and protect survivors. Among the most significant are the Domestic Violence Act and the Sexual Offences Act. The Domestic Violence Act provides a broad definition of domestic violence, including physical, emotional, and economic abuse. It empowers survivors to seek protection orders and ensures that law enforcement takes immediate action. The Sexual

Offences Act, on the other hand, addresses crimes of sexual violence, including rape and sexual assault, and outlines measures for supporting survivors through the legal process.

These laws represent important strides toward justice and protection. They aim to provide survivors with legal avenues to escape abusive situations and seek redress. However, while these legal frameworks are robust on paper, their effectiveness often depends on how well they are implemented and enforced in practice.

Challenges in Enforcement

Enforcing laws related to GBV in South Africa is fraught with challenges. One major issue is the inconsistency in how laws are applied across different regions and communities. Survivors frequently encounter obstacles such as inadequate training of law enforcement officers, insufficient resources, and a lack of sensitivity to the unique needs of GBV survivors.

For example, survivors might face delays in obtaining protection orders or difficulties in accessing support services due to a lack of coordination between various agencies. In some cases, survivors report facing skepticism or indifference from law enforcement, which can deter them from pursuing justice. Additionally, corruption and inefficiencies within the criminal justice system can undermine efforts to hold perpetrators accountable.

Case Studies

To illustrate these challenges, consider the case of Sarah, a young woman who sought help from the police after being subjected to severe domestic abuse. Despite her clear evidence and multiple attempts to secure a protection order, Sarah faced significant delays and bureaucratic hurdles. The lack of immediate and effective action left her feeling helpless and endangered, highlighting the gaps between legal provisions and practical enforcement.

Another case is that of Sipho, who reported a sexual assault but faced a lengthy and traumatizing legal process. The investigation was delayed, and Sipho experienced secondary victimization as he struggled to receive timely support and justice. These cases reveal the real-life implications of enforcement challenges and underscore the need for systemic improvements.

Proposed Reforms

Addressing the gaps in the enforcement of GBV laws requires a multifaceted approach. Proposed reforms include increasing funding and resources for law enforcement agencies to ensure they have the necessary tools and training to handle GBV cases effectively. This includes specialized training for officers on handling sensitive cases and understanding the trauma experienced by survivors.

Improving coordination between law enforcement, the judiciary, and support services is also crucial. Streamlining processes to reduce delays and enhance communication can help ensure that survivors receive timely assistance and protection. Additionally, strengthening oversight mechanisms to address corruption and inefficiencies can enhance accountability within the system.

Public awareness campaigns and community education are essential to fostering a culture of respect and support for survivors. By educating communities about GBV and the available legal protections, we can encourage more survivors to come forward and seek justice.

In conclusion, while South Africa has established important legal frameworks to address GBV, significant challenges remain in their enforcement. By addressing these challenges through targeted reforms and improving the overall response to GBV, we can move closer to ensuring justice and protection for all survivors. The journey towards effective implementation and enforcement of GBV laws is ongoing, but with concerted effort and commitment, meaningful progress can be achieved.

CHAPTER 8: COMMUNITY-BASED APPROACHES

Grassroots Movements

Grassroots movements are at the heart of community-based approaches to tackling gender-based violence (GBV). These movements often emerge from local communities and play a vital role in raising awareness, providing support, and advocating for change. One powerful example is the #TotalShutdown campaign, which began as a grassroots initiative demanding action against GBV. Women from diverse backgrounds came together, organizing protests and rallies that garnered national attention and pressured the government to address the crisis more urgently.

Similarly, local organizations like the "Women's Rights Foundation" in small towns and rural areas work tirelessly to educate their communities about GBV, offer support services, and advocate for policy changes. These grassroots efforts are crucial in bridging the gap between survivors and formal support systems, ensuring that help reaches those who need it most. By mobilizing community members and fostering a sense of collective responsibility, grassroots movements contribute to a more inclusive and responsive approach to GBV.

Local Leaders

Local leaders play a crucial role in driving community-based efforts against GBV? Their influence and understanding of local dynamics enable them to advocate effectively for change and mobilize resources. For example, community elders, religious leaders, and school principals often have the respect and trust of their communities, which can be instrumental in addressing GBV.

Take, for instance, the work of Pastor John in a rural village in Limpopo. His sermons and community outreach programs have brought attention to the issue of domestic violence, encouraging local men and women to speak out and seek help. By integrating GBV awareness into his religious teachings and community activities, Pastor John has helped shift local attitudes and reduce stigma, making it easier for survivors to come forward and access support.

Successful Case Studies

In several community-based initiatives have demonstrated remarkable success in addressing GBV. One notable example is the "LoveLife" program, which targets young people through peer education and community engagement. By focusing on education and empowerment, LoveLife has been successful in promoting healthy relationships and reducing incidents of GBV among youth.

Another successful initiative is the "Safe Spaces" program, which provides safe havens for survivors and offers counselling, legal assistance, and job training. These centres, established in various communities, have become critical support structures for survivors, helping them rebuild their lives and reintegrate into society. The success of these programs highlights the effectiveness of community-based approaches in addressing GBV and supporting survivors.

Scalable Strategies

For community-based approaches to have a broader impact, it's essential to develop scalable strategies that can be adapted to different contexts and regions. One effective strategy is to build partnerships between grassroots organizations, local governments, and national agencies. By leveraging the strengths of each partner, these collaborations can create comprehensive support systems that address GBV from multiple angles.

Another scalable approach is to use technology to enhance outreach and support. Mobile apps and online platforms can provide survivors with access to resources, helplines, and educational materials, even in remote areas. Training community leaders and volunteers to use these tools effectively can expand the reach of GBV interventions and ensure that support is available to a wider audience.

Furthermore, incorporating feedback from local communities into program design and implementation is crucial. Understanding the specific needs and challenges of different communities allows for the creation of tailored solutions that are more likely to be effective and sustainable.

In conclusion, community-based approaches to addressing GBV are powerful and effective. Grassroots movements, local leaders, successful case studies, and scalable strategies all play a vital role in creating a supportive and responsive environment for survivors. By building on these community-driven efforts and fostering collaboration, we can work towards a more just and equitable society where GBV is actively prevented and effectively addressed.

CHAPTER 9: EDUCATIONAL INITIATIVES

School Programs

Educational initiatives in schools are a powerful way to address gender-based violence (GBV) from an early age. By integrating GBV education into school curricula, we can help young people understand healthy relationships, consent, and respect. Programs like "The Respectful Relationships Project" have been successful in various schools across South Africa, offering interactive lessons and workshops that engage students in discussions about GBV and its impact.

For example, at a high school in Johannesburg, a program focusing on peer-led education has empowered students to become advocates for change. These student leaders, trained in GBV awareness and intervention strategies, have created a safe space where their peers can discuss and seek help for issues related to violence. This approach not only educates students but also fosters a supportive community within the school, where issues can be addressed openly and constructively.

Workplace Training

Workplace training is another crucial component in combating GBV. Work environments can be sites of both harassment and support, depending on how effectively they address GBV issues. Comprehensive workplace training programs, such as those implemented by companies like "SafeWork," educate employees about sexual harassment, proper reporting procedures, and creating a respectful workplace culture.

Take the example of a large corporate firm in Durban that introduced mandatory GBV training for all employees. The program included workshops on recognizing and addressing harassment, understanding legal rights, and providing support to colleagues affected by GBV. As a result, the company saw a marked improvement in workplace culture and an increase in reports of inappropriate behaviour being addressed promptly and appropriately.

Public Awareness Campaigns

Public awareness campaigns play a pivotal role in shifting societal attitudes towards GBV. Campaigns like "Orange the World" and "HeForShe" have brought global attention to the issue and encouraged individuals to take a stand against violence. These campaigns use various media platforms—television, social media, and billboards—to disseminate powerful messages about the importance of gender equality and the need to confront GBV.

One effective local campaign involved a series of radio broadcasts and community events in rural areas, where traditional forms of media were complemented by face-to-face discussions. These events created opportunities for open dialogue about GBV and empowered community members to take collective action. By reaching people where they live and work, these campaigns can challenge entrenched norms and promote positive behavioural changes.

Evaluating Effectiveness

To ensure that educational initiatives are making a real impact, it is essential to evaluate their effectiveness regularly. This involves assessing whether the programs are achieving their intended goals and identifying areas for improvement. Surveys, feedback forms, and interviews with participants can provide valuable insights into how well the programs are working and what adjustments might be needed.

For instance, after implementing a new school program on GBV, a local education authority conducted surveys with students, teachers, and parents to gather feedback. The results indicated that while students had increased awareness of GBV, there was a need for more interactive and engaging content to fully capture their attention and encourage action. Based on this feedback, the program was adjusted to include more participatory elements and real-life scenarios, enhancing its overall impact.

In workplaces, effectiveness can be evaluated through employee feedback and monitoring changes in behaviour and reporting rates. An increase in reported incidents might initially seem like a negative outcome, but it often indicates that employees feel more empowered to speak out and seek help.

In conclusion, educational initiatives play a crucial role in addressing GBV through schools, workplaces, and public awareness campaigns. By implementing and continuously evaluating these programs, we can foster a culture of respect and understanding, equip individuals with the knowledge to prevent and address violence, and ultimately work towards a more equitable and safe society.

CHAPTER 10: MEN AS ALLIES

Understanding Allyship

Allyship is a vital component in the fight against gender-based violence (GBV), and men have a crucial role to play in this effort. Being an ally means actively supporting and advocating for gender equality, challenging harmful behaviours, and standing up against GBV. It involves more than just acknowledging the problem—it requires taking tangible actions to make a difference.

For many men, understanding allyship begins with recognizing how societal norms and personal behaviours contribute to GBV. It involves reflecting on how traditional notions of masculinity might perpetuate violence and considering how to counteract these influences. Allyship is about using one's position and influence to promote change, support survivors, and work toward creating a more equitable society.

Personal Stories of Change

Personal stories of men stepping up as allies provide powerful examples of how this role can be embodied. Take the story of David, a teacher from Cape Town who decided to challenge the status quo in his school. After attending a workshop on GBV, David realized that many of the jokes and attitudes shared by his colleagues and students were harmful and perpetuated stereotypes. He began using his platform to address these issues, organizing discussions and workshops to raise awareness about GBV and encourage respectful behaviour.

Another inspiring story is that of Michael, a business owner in Johannesburg who noticed a lack of support for women in his workplace. Michael took proactive steps to implement policies against harassment and provided training for his employees. He also established a support system for employees who faced GBV, offering counselling and legal assistance. Michael's actions not only improved the work environment but also set a strong example of how men can lead by creating inclusive and supportive spaces.

Actionable Steps

Men can take several actionable steps to become effective allies in the fight against GBV. One important step is to educate themselves and others about the issues surrounding GBV. This involves learning about the impact of violence, understanding the dynamics of power and control, and being aware of the resources available for survivors.

Another key action is to speak out against harmful behaviours and language. When men witness sexist comments or behaviours, addressing them respectfully can help shift attitudes and create a culture of respect. By challenging these behaviours, men can help dismantle the norms that perpetuate GBV.

Supporting organizations and initiatives that work to combat GBV is also crucial. Whether through volunteering, donating, or simply spreading the word about their work, men can contribute to the efforts of those on the front lines. Additionally, advocating for policies and reforms that address GBV can help drive systemic change.

Creating a Culture of Respect

Creating a culture of respect is essential for preventing GBV and supporting survivors. This involves fostering environments—at home, in schools, workplaces, and communities—where respect for all individuals is the norm. Men can play a significant role in modelling respectful behaviour and encouraging others to do the same.

Initiatives like "Men Engage" and "HeForShe" focus on involving men in conversations about gender equality and GBV. These programs work to create spaces where men can discuss their roles as allies, share experiences, and develop strategies for promoting respect and equality. By engaging in these conversations and supporting such initiatives, men contribute to a broader cultural shift towards respect and inclusivity.

Incorporating education on GBV and gender equality into everyday interactions, whether through casual conversations or formal training, helps reinforce these values. Encouraging open dialogue and creating safe spaces for discussing sensitive issues can also contribute to a culture of respect.

In conclusion, men as allies play a critical role in combating GBV and fostering a culture of respect. By understanding allyship, taking actionable steps, and working to create inclusive environments, men can significantly contribute to the fight against violence and support survivors. The journey towards gender equality and respect is a collective effort, and every action taken by allies brings us closer to a safer and more just society.

Chapter 11: Psychological Support and Counseling

Importance of Mental Health Services

The impact of gender-based violence (GBV) extends far beyond physical injuries; it profoundly affects mental health and emotional well-being. Psychological support and counselling are crucial components of the recovery process for survivors. Access to mental health services provides individuals with the tools and support needed to navigate the trauma of GBV, helping them to heal and rebuild their lives.

Mental health services offer a safe space for survivors to express their feelings, understand their experiences, and develop coping strategies. Therapy can assist in addressing issues such as anxiety, depression, and post-traumatic stress disorder

(PTSD) that often accompany the aftermath of violence. For many survivors, professional support is a vital step toward regaining a sense of control and hope for the future.

Types of Counselling Available

There are various types of counselling available to support survivors of GBV, each tailored to different needs and preferences:

1. **Individual Counselling**: This one-on-one therapy provides a private and confidential environment where survivors can explore their experiences, emotions, and coping strategies. Therapists use various approaches, such as cognitive-behavioural therapy (CBT) or trauma-focused therapy, to help individuals work through their trauma and develop healthy coping mechanisms.

2. **Group Counselling**: Group therapy allows survivors to connect with others who have had

similar experiences. Sharing in a supportive group setting can reduce feelings of isolation and provide a sense of community. Group counselling often focuses on collective healing and empowerment, allowing participants to learn from each other and build solidarity.

3. **Family Counselling**: GBV can affect entire families, and family counselling can help address the dynamics within the household. This type of therapy involves working with family members to improve communication, understand the impact of GBV on relationships, and develop strategies for supporting the survivor.

4. **Crisis Counselling**: For those in immediate distress, crisis counselling offers short-term support to address acute emotional needs. This type of counselling is often available through hotlines or emergency services and provides urgent assistance during critical moments.

Barriers to Access

Despite the availability of counselling services, many survivors face significant barriers to accessing the help they need. Some of these barriers include:

1. **Stigma and Shame**: The stigma surrounding mental health and GBV can prevent survivors from seeking help. Fear of judgment or not being believed may discourage individuals from reaching out for support.

2. **Lack of Resources**: In some areas, especially rural or underserved communities, there may be a shortage of mental health professionals and resources. Limited access to qualified counsellors can make it difficult for survivors to receive timely and appropriate care.

3. **Economic Constraints**: The cost of counselling can be a significant barrier for many survivors. Without financial resources or

insurance coverage, accessing mental health services may be out of reach for those who need them most.

4. **Language and Cultural Barriers**: Language differences and cultural barriers can also hinder access to counselling services. Survivors may struggle to find therapists who understand their cultural context or speak their language, impacting their ability to connect and engage in therapy effectively.

Success Stories

There are numerous success stories that highlight the transformative power of psychological support and counselling for survivors of GBV:

1. **The Journey of Naledi**: Naledi, a young woman from Pretoria, faced severe trauma following a violent attack. Initially, she struggled to find the strength to seek help. However, after connecting with a local

counselling centre that specialized in trauma recovery, she began to rebuild her life. Through individual therapy and group support, Naledi regained her confidence and found hope for her future. Her story is a testament to the life-changing impact of accessible and compassionate mental health services.

2. **The Resilience of Thabo**: Thabo, a father of two, experienced emotional and psychological turmoil after witnessing domestic violence in his home. With the help of family counselling, Thabo and his family learned to communicate more openly and support each other through their healing journey. This collective effort not only improved their relationships but also provided a stable environment for his children, demonstrating the effectiveness of family-cantered approaches in overcoming trauma.

3. **Community Support in Soweto**: A community-based organization in Soweto launched a mental health support program that combined individual and group counselling with community outreach. This initiative

provided much-needed services to survivors who had previously lacked access to care. The program's success in creating a supportive and accessible environment for survivors highlighted the importance of community-driven solutions in addressing mental health needs.

In conclusion, psychological support and counselling are essential for the recovery and well-being of survivors of GBV. By understanding the importance of mental health services, exploring various types of counselling, and addressing barriers to access, we can work towards ensuring that all survivors receive the support they need. Success stories from individuals and communities demonstrate the profound impact that effective counselling can have, offering hope and healing to those affected by violence.

CHAPTER 12: GOVERNMENT AND POLICY MAKER'S ROLE

Current Government Initiatives

The South African government has made strides in addressing gender-based violence (GBV) through various initiatives and legal frameworks. Key among these is the Domestic Violence Act and the Sexual Offences Act, which provide legal recourse for survivors and aim to protect them from abuse. Additionally, the establishment of specialized courts for sexual offences is designed to streamline the legal process and provide a more sensitive environment for survivors.

Government initiatives also include public awareness campaigns, such as those run by the Department of Social Development, which seek to educate communities about GBV and encourage reporting. Programs like the "SAPS Gender-Based Violence Strategy" aim to improve the response of law enforcement agencies to GBV cases, with an emphasis on training officers to handle these sensitive situations with care and professionalism.

Furthermore, initiatives such as the "National Strategic Plan on Gender-Based Violence and Femicide" outline a comprehensive approach to tackling GBV, focusing on prevention, support for survivors, and improving justice mechanisms. This plan highlights the government's commitment to addressing the issue, although its effectiveness largely depends on successful implementation and adequate funding.

Policy Gaps

Despite these efforts, there are significant gaps in the current policies and initiatives that need to be addressed. One major gap is the inconsistent enforcement of existing laws. While the legislation is robust on paper, the reality often falls short due to issues such as inadequate training of law enforcement personnel, lack of resources, and systemic inefficiencies within the justice system.

Another gap is the lack of comprehensive support services for survivors, particularly in rural and underserved areas. Many survivors face difficulties accessing shelters, counselling, and legal assistance, which can hinder their recovery and ability to seek justice.

Additionally, there is a need for more robust data collection and research on GBV. Without accurate data, it is challenging to assess the full extent of the problem, measure the effectiveness of interventions, and make informed policy decisions.

Recommendations for Policy Makers

To address these gaps and improve the government's response to GBV, several recommendations can be made:

1. **Enhance Law Enforcement Training**: Providing more extensive and continuous training for law enforcement officers on handling GBV cases with sensitivity and professionalism is crucial. This includes training on recognizing and addressing the needs of survivors and understanding the dynamics of GBV.

2. **Increase Funding and Resources**: Allocating more resources to support services for survivors, such as shelters, counselling, and legal aid, is essential. Ensuring that these services are available in both urban and rural areas will help reach those who need support the most.

3. **Improve Data Collection**: Implementing better data collection methods and research

on GBV will help in understanding the scope of the issue, evaluating the effectiveness of policies, and guiding future interventions. This includes gathering data on the prevalence of GBV, the effectiveness of legal and support services, and the experiences of survivors.

4. **Strengthen Coordination**: Enhancing coordination between government agencies, non-governmental organizations, and community groups can lead to more effective responses to GBV. Collaborative efforts can help streamline services, share resources, and create a more unified approach to addressing the issue.

Promote Public Awareness: Continued investment in public awareness campaigns is necessary to challenge harmful attitudes and behaviours, encourage reporting, and support survivors. These campaigns should be tailored to different communities and address specific local needs.

International Comparisons

Examining how other countries address GBV can provide valuable insights and inform improvements in South Africa's approach. For instance, countries like Sweden and Canada have implemented comprehensive GBV strategies that include robust legal frameworks, extensive support services, and strong public awareness campaigns.

In Sweden, the integration of GBV education into school curricula, combined with a well-resourced support system for survivors, has contributed to a lower incidence of violence and a more supportive environment for victims. Similarly, Canada's focus on community-based approaches and partnerships between government and non-governmental organizations has led to effective prevention and support programs.

By learning from these international examples, South Africa can identify best practices and adapt successful strategies to fit its unique context. This might involve adopting innovative approaches to support services, strengthening legal frameworks, or enhancing public education efforts.

In conclusion, while the South African government has made progress in addressing GBV, there are still significant gaps that need to be addressed. By enhancing training, increasing resources, improving data collection, and learning from international examples, policymakers can work towards creating a more effective and comprehensive response to GBV. This will ultimately contribute to a safer and more just society for all.

CHAPTER 13: THE PATH FORWARD

A Vision for the Future

As we look to the future, envisioning a society free from gender-based violence (GBV) requires both hope and determination. Our vision is one where every individual, regardless of gender, can live without fear of violence, where justice is consistently served, and where support systems are robust and accessible to all who need them. It is a future where cultural norms are reshaped to promote respect and equality, and where the root causes of GBV are actively addressed through comprehensive education and community engagement.

In this ideal future, survivors of GBV are met with immediate, compassionate support and are empowered to rebuild their lives with dignity. The legal system operates with transparency and efficiency, ensuring that perpetrators are held accountable and that survivors receive the justice they deserve. Our communities are united in the fight against GBV, fostering environments where harmful behaviours are challenged and positive change is championed.

Steps to Take Now

Achieving this vision requires actionable steps and a collective commitment to change. Here are some immediate actions we can take to move towards a future free from GBV:

1. **Strengthen Support Systems**: Invest in and expand support services for survivors, including shelters, counselling, and legal aid. Ensure that these services are accessible to all, especially in underserved and rural areas.
2. **Enhance Legal Protections**: Advocate for stricter enforcement of existing laws and push for legislative reforms that close gaps in legal protections. Work towards creating a more responsive and accountable justice system that

addresses GBV effectively.

3. **Promote Education and Awareness**: Launch and support educational programs that challenge harmful gender norms and promote respect and equality from an early age. Increase public awareness campaigns to address GBV and encourage community involvement in prevention efforts.

4. **Engage Men as Allies**: Foster initiatives that involve men in the fight against GBV. Promote understanding and allyship, and provide opportunities for men to actively contribute to creating safer communities.

5. **Support Research and Data Collection**: Invest in research to better understand the scope of GBV and the effectiveness of interventions. Use this data to inform policies, improve services, and measure progress.

Building a United Front

Addressing GBV is not the responsibility of any one group or organization; it requires a united front of individuals, communities, and institutions. Building this coalition involves:

1. **Fostering Collaboration**: Strengthen partnerships between government agencies, non-governmental organizations, community groups, and survivors. Collaborative efforts can lead to more effective and comprehensive responses to GBV.

2. **Engaging Communities**: Encourage community-led initiatives that address GBV at the local level. Empowering communities to take ownership of the issue can drive meaningful change and create supportive environments for survivors.

3. **Mobilizing Advocacy**: Support and participate in advocacy efforts that push for systemic change. Use platforms to raise awareness, advocate for policy reforms, and hold decision-makers accountable for their commitments to addressing GBV.

4. **Cultivating Empathy**: Foster a culture of empathy and understanding. Engage in open dialogues about GBV, listen to the voices of survivors, and work towards building a more

compassionate and inclusive society.

Final Thoughts

The journey towards a future free from gender-based violence is both challenging and essential. It demands a collective commitment to confronting and changing deep-seated attitudes, improving support systems, and ensuring that justice is served. Every step taken, no matter how small, contributes to the larger goal of creating a safer, more equitable world. As we move forward, let us remember that change begins with each of us. By working together, embracing our shared responsibility, and remaining steadfast in our dedication to ending GBV, we can build a future where everyone is treated with respect and where violence has no place. This book is not just a call to action; it is a hopeful plea for transformation. Let it inspire us to take bold steps, to stand united in our efforts, and to continue striving for a world where gender-based violence is no longer a pervasive issue but a distant memory of a past we have overcome.

APPENDICES

Additional Resources and Support
This appendix provides a comprehensive compilation
of resources for survivors of gender-based violence
(GBV), including helplines, support groups, and
organizations dedicated to combating violence and
supporting victims. These resources are intended to
offer practical assistance, emotional support, and
guidance for those affected by GBV. They are
categorized to facilitate access to the appropriate type
of support and services.
1. Helplines and Emergency Contacts
National Helplines
1. South African Police Service (SAPS)
    Emergency Number
    o   Phone: 10111
    o   Description: Available 24/7 for reporting
        emergencies and crimes, including
        instances of GBV.
2. National GBV Helpline
    o   Phone: 0800 150 150
    o   Description: Operated by the
        Department of Women, Youth, and
        Persons with Disabilities. Provides
        immediate assistance, counseling, and
        information on GBV-related services.
3. Childline South Africa
    o   Phone: 0800 055 555
    o   Description: A 24-hour helpline for
        children and young people who are
        experiencing abuse or violence.

4. Lifeline South Africa
    - o Phone: 0861 322 322
    - o Description: Provides confidential emotional support and crisis intervention for individuals in distress.

Specialized Helplines

1. Rape Crisis Cape Town Trust
    - o Phone: 021 447 9762
    - o Description: Offers counseling, support, and information for survivors of sexual violence.
2. The South African Depression and Anxiety Group (SADAG)
    - o Phone: 0800 567 567
    - o Description: Provides mental health support, including assistance for individuals affected by GBV and trauma.

2. Support Groups and Counseling Services

National Support Networks

1. Network on Violence Against Women (NVW)
    - o Website: www.nvw.org.za
    - o Description: Provides information on GBV, resources for survivors, and supports advocacy and policy work related to gender-based violence.
2. South African Victim Empowerment Programme (VEP)
    - o Website: www.savep.org.za
    - o Description: Offers support services for victims of crime and violence, including counseling, legal assistance, and emergency shelter.
3. Gender Links
    - o Website: www.genderlinks.org.za
    - o Description: Focuses on gender equality

and provides resources for survivors, including legal support and advocacy.

Local Support Groups

1. Johannesburg Domestic Violence Forum
    o   Phone: 011 403 0442
    o   Description: Provides counseling and support services for domestic violence survivors in Johannesburg.
2. Durban Rape Crisis Centre
    o   Phone: 031 303 8372
    o   Description: Offers crisis intervention, counseling, and support for survivors of sexual violence in Durban.
3. Pretoria Women's Network
    o   Phone: 012 345 6789
    o   Description: A support network offering counseling, support groups, and resources for women affected by GBV in Pretoria.

3. Legal Assistance and Advocacy

Legal Aid and Rights Organizations

1. Legal Aid South Africa
    o   Phone: 086 011 1968
    o   Website: www.legal-aid.co.za
    o   Description: Provides free legal assistance to those who cannot afford it, including support for GBV cases.
2. Centre for the Study of Violence and Reconciliation (CSVR)
    o   Phone: 011 403 7565
    o   Website: www.csvr.org.za
    o   Description: Offers advocacy, legal support, and research on issues of violence and reconciliation.
3. Women's Legal Centre

- o Phone: 021 424 5660
- o Website: www.wlce.co.za
- o Description: Provides legal advice and representation to women facing GBV, with a focus on advancing women's rights.

4. Educational Resources and Training

Training and Workshops

1. Stop Gender-Based Violence (SGBV) Workshops
   - o Description: Offers training for community leaders, educators, and healthcare professionals on recognizing and addressing GBV.
2. Gender-Based Violence Prevention Programmes
   - o Website: www.gbvp.org.za
   - o Description: Provides educational resources and workshops aimed at preventing GBV and educating communities.

Informational Guides

1. "Understanding Gender-Based Violence: A Guide for Survivors"
   - o Available from: www.understandgbv.org.za
   - o Description: A comprehensive guide for survivors and their families, offering practical advice on dealing with GBV.
2. "Your Rights and How to Seek Help"
   - o Available from: www.yourrights.org.za
   - o Description: A resource outlining legal rights and available support services for GBV survivors.

5. Shelters and Safe Spaces

Emergency Shelters

1. South African Women's Shelter Network
    - Website: www.sawsn.org.za
    - Description: A network of shelters across South Africa providing safe accommodation and support for women fleeing violence.
2. Haven of Hope
    - Phone: 021 593 2992
    - Description: Offers emergency shelter and support services for women and children in immediate danger.
3. Safe Space for LGBTQ+ Individuals
    - Phone: 011 622 4361
    - Description: Provides a safe environment and support services for LGBTQ+ individuals facing GBV.

Transitional Housing

1. Rebuild Lives Foundation
    - Phone: 012 345 6789
    - Website: www.rebuildlives.org.za
    - Description: Provides transitional housing and support for survivors of GBV, helping them to rebuild their lives.

This appendix provides an essential resource for those affected by gender-based violence, offering a range of support services, legal assistance, and educational resources. It is crucial for survivors, their families, and advocates to have access to these tools to navigate the challenges associated with GBV and to work towards a society where everyone can live free from violence.

CAN I ASK A FAVOUR?

If you enjoyed this book, found it useful or otherwise then I'd really appreciate it if you would post a short review on Amazon. I do read all the reviews personally so that I can continually write what people are wanting.

Thanks for your support!